DIET COOKBOOK FOR CHRONIC FATIGUE

The Best Foods to Eat If You Have CFS

HALEA GREENE

Table of Contents

CHAPTER ONE

INFATIGUE DIET FOR CHRONIC FATIGUE

The Best Foods to Eat If You Have CFS

If you have chronic fatigue syndrome (CFS) or myalgic encephalomyelitis (ME/CFS), it's important to follow a specific diet. It's not possible to cure chronic fatigue syndrome with diet alone, but you can help yourself feel better by increasing your energy and addressing any nutrient deficiencies you may be experiencing.

Foods and beverages that may be aggravating your symptoms should be avoided in the context of a chronic fatigue syndrome diet. What works best for you will take some trial and error, and that begins with learning as much as possible about how food might be affecting your symptoms.

Benefits

Many studies on chronic fatigue syndrome diet and nutrition are inconclusive, and the studies that are available are of poor quality. Chronic inflammation has been linked to ME/CFS. There hasn't been any research done on the effects of an anti-inflammatory diet on this condition. Patients with this condition may benefit from it because it is generally regarded as a healthy diet.

Many people with ME/CFS are deficient in vitamins, minerals, and essential fatty acids, according to a 2017 review of nutritional treatments for chronic fatigue syndrome published in Biomedicine & Pharmacotherapy.

1

Nutritional deficiencies that may be contributing to the symptoms of ME/CFS can be corrected by following a well-balanced chronic fatigue syndrome diet. If necessary, dietary supplements can be beneficial.

Certain nutrients found in foods may help alleviate fatigue and other symptoms, according to a review of diet and supplement studies published in the Journal of Nutrition and Human Dietetics in 2017.

2 Among them were:

NAD+ hydrochloride of Nicotinamide (NADH)

• Probiotics

• CoQ10

• Polyphenolics – (especially from chocolate with a high cocoa content)

Chocolate contains polyphenols, an antioxidant that may be particularly beneficial for those suffering from chronic fatigue syndrome. Polyphenols in dark chocolate have been shown to reduce the symptoms of ME/CFS, according to one study. Polyphenols can also be found in foods such as green tea, berries, and legumes. However, they haven't been studied in detail for this purpose.

Antioxidants such as polyphenols and others are thought to repair damage to molecules that can result in disease. In one theory about the causes of chronic fatigue syndrome, free radicals overwhelm the body due to oxidative stress, and antioxidants counteract this process.

Free radicals: What Are They and Why Do They Matter?

Supplementing with either D-ribose or omega-3 fatty acids has also been shown to reduce some of the symptoms of ME/CFS.

4

Since low levels of many nutrients were found in people with chronic fatigue syndrome, many of these studies have focused on nutritional supplementation as a treatment option. If you want to increase your nutrient intake, it's best to start with food.

CHAPTER TWO

Angiogenesis and Chronic Fatigue Syndrome-Related Inflammation

Exactly How Does It Work?

It is the goal of the CFS diet to reduce fatigue, prevent nutrient deficiencies, and maintain inflammation under control through nutrition. There are no rules in this environment. To reduce inflammation-promoting chemicals in your body, eat foods that provide a steady supply of long-lasting energy and a healthier balance of fats and antioxidants. 1

Duration

You can and should stick to the chronic fatigue syndrome diet for the rest of your life, if you have this condition. Even if it helps your ME/CFS symptoms, it's a diet that's good for your overall health as well. 4

What to Eat!

Foods That Meet Government Standards

• Foodstuffs that are in season (any, especially berries)

• Fruits and Vegetables (any, especially leafy greens and orange-colored options)

Beans and other legumes that have been dried

Cracked or whole grains

• Seafood and fish

Whole soy foods (e.g., tofu or tempeh)

Fermentation of dairy products (e.g., yogurt or kefir)

Avocado, olive oil, nuts, and seeds are excellent sources of healthy fats, as are

• Chocolate that is very dark in color (in moderation)

• Herbs and spices (fresh or dried)

Foods That Aren't In Compliance

Fast food and fried food are two examples of this category.

• Meals in a bag or a freezer

• Snacks in a can

Soft drinks with added sugar

•   Foods that contain added sugar or white flour, such as cookies and cakes.

Oils containing omega-6 fats, like margarine,

• Alcohol

• Caffeine

There is no one-size-fits-all diet for chronic fatigue syndrome, and tailoring a healthy eating plan to your individual needs will help you stick to it. Rather than following a rigid diet, this approach relies on a variety of whole foods at each meal and snack to achieve a nutritionally complete diet.

The Most Effective Alternatives

Fruits like berries, cherries, and apples are particularly high in polyphenols. The polyphenols in dark chocolate have been shown to have health benefits, so including it in your diet may be worthwhile. 3

Antioxidant-rich vegetables, like red or orange vegetables such as carrots and sweet potatoes, should be incorporated into your diet as many times a week. Cooking enhances some nutrients, while eating them raw preserves fiber and other nutrients. A good mix of cooked and raw foods is ideal.

Salmon, mackerel, and sardines are particularly high in omega-3 fats, which have been shown to reduce inflammation, making them excellent sources of lean protein.

5

For nuts, walnuts come out on top with flax seeds (or flax meal, which is easier to digest), chia seeds (also known as hulled hemp seeds), and hemp seed (also known as hulled hemp seeds).

Probiotics can be found in fermented dairy products like kefir and Greek yogurt. They help maintain a healthy digestive system, but they also provide a food source for probiotics, which may help alleviate your symptoms. 6

Unsaturated fats, such as those found in olive oil, olives, avocados, and all nuts and seeds, have been shown to reduce inflammation.

• Chocolate: Dark chocolate is a good source of polyphenols; however, milk chocolate bars and chocolate desserts should be avoided.

Foods You Should Avoid

Pro-inflammatory omega-6 fats like corn, soybean, and other vegetable oils are commonly found in snack foods and packaged meals.

7

Adding sugar and white flour to foods like desserts and white bread can lead to the production of cytokines, which can cause inflammation in the body.

CHAPTER THREE

8

If you're already exhausted, caffeine and alcohol may increase your cortisol levels, which can exacerbate your symptoms. Use them sparingly and keep in mind that they may exacerbate symptoms of ME/CFS because of the paucity of research on their impact on this condition.

All-Natural Foods Diets

Besides these pro-inflammatory foods, there may be foods that do not agree with you due to an intolerance or allergy. ' Could an elimination diet work? Keep a food and symptom journal to spot any patterns and help you narrow down the list of foods to avoid.

If certain foods make you feel worse, talk to your doctor about getting tested. The results of a 2012 study on the dietary habits of people with chronic fatigue syndrome found that rather than following one specific diet recommendation, people should make dietary changes based on

known allergies or intolerances.
9

Recommendation for a good time

There are no hard and fast rules about when you should eat, but if you don't skip meals and spread them out throughout the day, you may find that you have more energy. Aim for three meals a day at the very least, beginning with breakfast as soon as you awaken.

Fill up on healthy snacks like fruit and Greek yogurt with a few nuts when you're hungry in between meals. It's important to eat a variety of foods in order to keep you feeling full and energized until the next meal, such as fruits, vegetables, and healthy fats.

Tips and Tricks in the Kitchen

Avoid deep-frying your food by substituting extra virgin olive oil instead of corn or vegetable oil and using healthy cooking methods like sautéing, grilling, roasting, braising, or air-frying.

Slightly steaming your vegetables rather than boiling them helps them retain a greater amount of nutritional value. In addition, the concentrated antioxidants found in herbs and spices encourage their liberal use.

Considerations

It's best to experiment with foods and see what works (or doesn't) for you until more research is done on the CFS diet. You should only make small dietary adjustments at a time in order to see how they affect your health. Even if the change is for the better, it could make your symptoms worse for a short period of time.

Make an appointment with your doctor or other healthcare professional before beginning any new supplement regimen.

10 As with any medication, some supplements may interact with other medications or have undesirable side effects.

When you make dietary changes, your body is able to function better and heal itself.

Try to be patient and focus on the task at hand at hand. Even if your symptoms don't improve, remember that many aspects of the chronic fatigue syndrome diet are good for your overall health.

Words

A healthy and balanced diet can support your body and make it work better so that you may feel better, regardless of whether you have chronic fatigue syndrome or another chronic health condition. A diet that is based on whole foods and allows you to make your own food choices is the best. Remember that fad diets and quick fixes are difficult to maintain and rarely work in the long term, so avoid them at all costs.

Living with Chronic Fatigue Syndrome: Tips for Success

In many ways, Myalgic encephalomyelitis/chronic fatigue syndrome (ME/CFS) will transform your life. It's a difficult condition to deal with.

However, there are steps you can take to make it less difficult.

You may have bad periods, or lapses, that are followed by better periods (remission). You'll be able to better manage your energy if you know what to expect.

Typical Day-to-Day Tasks

Simple morning rituals, like taking a shower, can be difficult when you're slipping back into your old habits. For tasks that are difficult for you, plan for additional time.

Take advantage of your newfound energy and get as much done as you can while you still have it. Try not to do it. The risk of a later crash increases the harder you push yourself. It's possible to relapse if you keep repeating this cycle.

No matter how long you've been in remission, maintaining a healthy work-life balance will be a constant challenge.

Exercise

ME/CFS sufferers may find it difficult to exercise because of their condition's limitations.

Individualized training plans are necessary because exhaustion can occur with any form of exercise. Establish a starting point for your exercise regimen with the help of your doctor or a physical therapist, and work your way up from there. Working past your limits without experiencing post-exercise fatigue is possible with this method (post-exertional malaise or PEM).

If your symptoms worsen as a result of your exercise routine, reduce your intensity back to the lowest level you could tolerate.

Your exercise regimen can be tweaked by a physical therapist. Take it easy. Proper timing is critical.

Nutrition

Manage your symptoms by keeping an eye on what you're eating. If you have a food or chemical sensitivity, stay away from it.

CHAPTER FOUR

Polyunsaturated and monounsaturated fats, as well as refined carbohydrates, have been found to be beneficial by many ME/CFS sufferers.

Consume a variety of small meals throughout the day. It's possible that eating four meals and three snacks a day keeps your energy levels high.

Nausea, which can accompany chronic fatigue syndrome, may be lessened by eating more frequently but in smaller portions. The following items should also be avoided in order to keep your energy levels in check:

- Sugar

- Sweeteners

- Alcohol

- Caffeine

Memory Enhancement

Some ME/CFS sufferers experience memory loss. To stay on top of your schedule and remember what needs to be done, use a day planner (either a paper one or a smartphone app).

When it's time to go somewhere or do something, set a reminder on your smartphone. Organize your thoughts by making to-do lists. Take a few "sticky notes."

Keep your brain active and sharpen your memory by

playing puzzles, word games, and card games, all of which can be found on your smartphone.

Work

A little more than half of those who suffer from ME/CFS are employed. It is possible that you may be eligible for disability benefits under the Americans with Disabilities Act (ADA). "Reasonable accommodations" must be provided by some employers to help disabled workers perform their duties.

Having a flexible work schedule, a place to rest, and written instructions for people with memory issues may be necessary for you. Workplace accommodations are based on how symptoms and your job performance are intertwined.

To qualify for disability benefits from either a private insurance policy or the Social Security Administration, you must be unable to work because of your condition.

Relationships

Coworkers, friends, family members and loved ones may struggle to comprehend ME/CFS. The impact on your day-to-day activities may be underestimated by them. Or, they may simply be unable to accept its validity. Friends and coworkers of those suffering from ME/CFS should be made aware of the illness.

Your personal relationships can be affected by chronic fatigue. Pain, fatigue, and medication side effects can limit your ability to participate in social activities, spend time with your children, or engage in sexual relations that are both healthy and fulfilling.

Seek Professional Guidance.

You may find that talking to other people who have the same condition helps you feel better. Support groups in your area can be found through referrals from your doctor.

Nearly one-half of all people with ME/CFS will go through periods of depressive illness. It's difficult to tell if you're depressed because some of the symptoms are similar to yours. Hopelessness, sadness, guilt, or worthlessness are all "red flags" for depression, and so are thoughts of suicide and death.

It is important to tell your doctor if you believe you are depressed. Depression treatments such as medication and therapy can alleviate both physical and psychological symptoms.

THE END